Too Soon

By: Marquita Johnson

©2011 Marquita Johnson. All rights reserved.
ISBN 978-1-105-31649-4

Preface

You always begin to think of the wrong things you do when it's too late. Why not be able to see into the future and know when you are going to do something wrong and think about it. It will never happen and we continue to do things wrong no matter how hard we try not to. Sometimes it seems like you can never stop doing the wrong things. It's like an impulse that makes you jump into something before you think. That's what happened to Shawn and Jazmean in their so-called relationship. They try to fix it, but it only gets worse.

Chapter 1

"Hey, Jazmean, let's go out tonight and have a little fun."

"I don't know if I'm going to like your idea of fun."

"Come on, Jazmean, we haven't had any *real* fun in months. Let's live a little! We have been together for four months."

"Shawn I have a job and you should have one, too, so I don't feel like going out to have *any* kind of fun."

"Fine, Jazmean, but you aren't going to spoil my fun."

"The only fun *you* need to be having is looking for a job so *you* can pay some bills."

"Look, I don't even want to go into that tonight. Why can't you just..."

"Just what, Shawn, work my ass off to support the both of us? You've got to be out of your mind if you're thinkin' that."

"You know what, if I find a job you will still be complaining."

The door slams and Jazmean is left with her thoughts while good old, 'Mr. Shawn', goes off to get drunk with no cares in the world. He's nothing but a low life, but Jazmean says she loves him and can help him. What a mistake that is. She is supporting the both of them on one job that pays six-fifty an hour. She is one strong individual to be only twenty-four.

"Hey, baby, I'm home."

"Let me guess...*still* with no job...that figures."

"Jazmean, I told you I just don't want to talk about that. Besides, it'll ruin my good night."

"What good night? The only good night I will ever see is the one when you come home from a job."

"Jazmean, I just..."

"You're just what, Shawn, you're just twenty-five and you can get a job anytime!"

"No, Jazmean I just love the way you take care of me."

"Well, get over it I'm not your momma, and I have to pay bills that *you* run up just sittin' in my apartment, soakin' up my air, eatin' my food, and watchin' my cable."

"So what are you trying to say, Jazmean?"

"I'm trying to say that until you get a job and learn something you can get out of my house!"

"But I don't..."

"And on top of that our relationship is over!"

The door slams and Shawn is left alone with the repercussions of what Jazmean said. 'Our relationship is over', just echoes in Shawn's head. He can't believe that after all of this time she would tell him something like that. With his determination to get his girl back he silently leaves the apartment to find a job.

"Shawn! What the hell are you doing?"

"What do you mean what am I doing? I'm getting ready for work."

"But why are you back in my house, in my kitchen, eatin' my food?"

"Look, Jazmean, I know what you said and I *am* taking you seriously. I just needed something to eat before I left."

"Well, next time let *me* know!"

"Okay! Now can I get a good-bye kiss?"

"I never gave you one before so why start now?"

"Really funny. I've got to go, so bye."

"Bye, Shawn."

"I can't believe it! He got a job!"

Jazmean was so surprised at what she saw right before her eyes, that she stumbled over the coffee table. She stands there frozen for at least a minute letting the whole thing soak in. Her man *finally* got himself together and all it took was an attitude from her. Now she felt like she was getting through to him. Don't speak *too soon*.

"Yo, Jazmean, are you home?"

"Yeah, Shawn, what's up?"

"Well, I have some bad news."

"What kind of bad news? Is it about your so-called job?"

"Now why you say it like that?"

"Because, you've lied once before and you obviously lied again."

"I swear to you I didn't lie. The bad news is that I have to work the night shift. That means I won't be able to see you as much."

"That's not bad news to me. I hardly see you anyway because you're always going off to some bar."

"Now, Jazmean, you know it's not like that at all. I just go have fun with my friends and I try to invite you, but *you* don't want to go."

"Look, why don't you just finish getting ready for work and get out of my house, Shawn."

"Oh, so it's like that now?"

"Yeah, it's like that."

Before you know it the apartment is quiet again and Jazmean is still getting over the shock of Shawn being in her apartment at seven-thirty in the morning when she kicked him out yesterday. She was happy that he had a job, no doubt, but it was still hard to believe that he had gotten one so quickly.

"It's about time you got here, Shawn!", a man in a leather suit said.

"Hey, what's up Marco, how is business going?"

"I hope it will be better with another runner like you to sell my product."

"I just have one question."

"I'm sure you do, Shawn, you're full of questions aren't you?"

"Well, Marco, I was wondering how long will it be before I start making the big money."

Marco hesitated to answer him because he was thinking he wouldn't make it past the first sell.

"Shawn, I'm gonna tell you like it is. If you make this first sell, and get me all my money on time, you will have at least half the profit by tomorrow."

"Yo, in that case give me the merchandise."

"Hold up, Big Man, we need to discuss a game plan. You're handling three kilos of my best chronic and we need to make sure that you get it all to the buyer without getting caught." Marco steps behind Shawn to look him over to see if he is really worthy of the job.

"Now Shawn, this is how this is going to go. The meeting place is down on 18th and Harlem. That's where a guy named 'T-Bone' will be. When he gives you the two grand that's when you give him the chronic. Are you gettin' this?" Shawn hesitates because he's thinking about what Jazmean is going to say when she finds out what his job is.

"Yeah man I got you."

"As I was saying, you give him the chronic and you leave. You don't communicate with him and he doesn't communicate with you. Now if you run into any trouble here's my nine. Just aim and shoot."

"Hold up, Marco, let's not take it that far. I'm sure I don't need a gun to deliver a little chronic to a customer."

Marco came real close to Shawn and said, "You never know who is there waiting to kill you, so you better be safe before you get sorry."

"I got you, man, I got you!"

Shawn leaves with the three kilos of chronic and the nine Marco gave him. All of a sudden he realizes he can't do it as easily as he thought he could. He thought to himself he couldn't just go back and say, "I'm chicken and I can't do this." He had to go give it a try. He stood in the hall going over the information that Marco had given him, and then left still thinking of Jazmean.

Shantell walks in the door of Jazmean's bookstore and looks around like she wants to buy something.

"Shantell, I don't know why *every* time you come in here you walk around like you want to buy something and you never do."

"Look, Jazmean, I would buy something if I thought it would be worth my time."

"You need to be buying a book on how to find a decent job that doesn't involve the taking off of clothes."

"Look, I am tired of you hatin' on my job like that. I strip and I am not ashamed of it." Jazmean gives Shantell a 'you ain't all that' look and continues to work.

"Well, I'll come by later, Jazmean, and maybe we can go out tonight and have some fun."

"I don't know about your kind of fun at those male strip joints."

"Oh, girl, you know you want to see someone else's behind besides Shawn's."

"Who said I've seen Shawn's behind?"

"You mean you haven't..."

"Yeah that's what I mean."

"Girl, I don't know what to say. You mean four months and nothing?"

"That's *exactly* what I mean."

"I got to go before I get to deep in your business."

Shantell left and Jazmean started thinking about what she had just said. '...Four months and nothing...' That's never crossed her mind until now. She tried to put it in the back of her mind so that she could do her work but it wasn't working. Now she began to realize *why* Shawn acted like he did. He hasn't had any in four months and it's her fault. Since she couldn't concentrate she closed the store up early and went home. When she got there she checked her messages.

"Beeeeep. Hi this is me, baby, I know you may not want to hear from me but I need to talk to you about something. I will see you around eight. Bye. Beeep." Now she regretted kicking him out of the apartment, but not enough to let him back in yet.

Riiiiiiiinnng.

"Hello."

"Hey, baby, it's me. How are you?"

"I'm fine, but I want to see you, Shawn. Can you come over?"

Shawn froze. He didn't know what to say. One minute she kicks him out and says he needs a job and then next she wants him to come to the apartment.

"Yes, Jazmean, I'll be there as soon as I can."

"Thank you, Shawn, it means a lot to me."

"I love you, too."

When Shawn hung up he knew something good was going to happen once he got to Jazmean's house. If he told her that he was selling drugs tonight it would ruin everything. He didn't

want to take that chance, so he just let it go.
"I guess I'll tell her tomorrow."

Chapter 2

Knock. Knock. Knock.

"Just a minute, I'm coming."

"Hey, baby, I'm here."

"Come in Shawn, I've been waiting for you."

When Shawn walked in the apartment he got the surprise he had been waiting for. Candles lit, music playing, and wonderful dinner on the table. The best thing was that Jazmean was dressed in the sexiest dress Shawn had ever seen. Shawn was so surprised he almost couldn't move.

"Damn, Jazmean, you look good tonight. I feel like I'm under dressed."

"That won't be a problem; I have your favorite suit waiting for you on the bed. Why don't you go take a shower and put it on while I finish preparing dinner."

"I think I'll do that, but don't you disappear on me."

"Don't worry I won't" Knock. Knock. Knock. "Go on I'll get the door, you just go get ready."

As he went into the bedroom Jazmean opened the door.

"Well, well, well, look who's all dressed up."

"I'm sorry, Shantell, I can't go out with you tonight I am staying in with Shawn."

"Are you finally going to give it up to him tonight?"

"Maybe. But that is not your business."

"Why not? You're going to tell me anyway, so why not now?"

"I think you better go before Shawn comes back out here and sees you."

"Let him see me!"

"Shantell, you *know* he doesn't like you so you *need* to leave."

"You will tell me what happens, right?"

"You know I will, Shantell, so go on and go party."

Jazmean closes the door and thinks about what Shantell said. "...You finally are going to give it up..." She stood there for at least a minute contemplating on if she was going to give it up to Shawn or not.

She stopped thinking long enough to finish dinner and put it on the table. By that time, Shawn had come out of the bedroom looking like a changed man.

"Now you look as good as I do."

"I could never look as good as you do right now, Jazmean, you are just *fine*."

"Well, thank you for that compliment. Shall we eat?"

"Yes, I think we should."

They walked over to the table hand in hand. Shawn was a gentleman and pulled out Jazmean's chair for her.

"The food looks really good", Shawn said, "When did you have the time to cook all of this?"

"I closed the store early and came home."

"Why?"

"Well, something someone said made me realize I should spend more time with you."

"Who ever told you that deserves a medal."

"That would only be if you knew who that person was."

"Well, who is it?"

"It's...Shantell."

"You mean to tell me that Shantell gave you the idea of spending time with *me* instead of going out with her to some strip club? I can't believe that girl would tell you to spend time with me, because we both hate each other."

"Now wait a minute, she doesn't hate you, you hate her."

"I don't really hate her, just the way she acts."

"Shawn, this is our night so let's stop talking about Shantell."

"I'm sorry for doing that, but I just can't help that I don't like her."

"Well, tonight you are going to forget about her and like me, because I am going to give you something that you won't forget."

"What will that be?"

"You will have to wait and find out after dinner."

"Well, in that case is it going to be dessert?" Jazmean looks at him with a sexy look that just gives him chills.

"Does that answer your question?"

"A lot better then you think. Let's eat, baby."

Shantell was kickin' it at the hottest male strip club in town. It was 'Hotties in Hizhouse.' She was trying to find her dream man. If she found him and he wasn't all that it would be a one-night stand. Most of all she wanted someone permanent. She was sick of just having a guy for one night. She wanted a lasting relationship with a man that she really liked. As she was walking she saw this fine dude standing over by the door. He was one of the bouncers and he looked like he would be a potential mate for her. She hesitated to walk over and talk to him but she got up the nerve.

"Hi. My name is Shantell. How are you this fine night?"

"I'm Jose and I'm fine. How about you?"

"I'm fine. I'm just having some fun. What are you doing after you leave here?"

"I might just go home and watch TV."

"Well, maybe we can get together."

She took a card out of her purse and wrote her number on it. She put it in his hand and closed it.

"Call me."

She walked away and went on about her business. Jose opens his hand and reads the card. It says: 'If you need a friend call me.' He smiled and put the number in his pocket. Shantell looked over at him and she could tell that he was interested in what she had to say.

Jazmean and Shawn were eating and talking to each other about what they wanted to do in their future. Shawn was just so surprised that he had so much in common with Jazmean. They hadn't just sat and had a conversation about each other since they first got together.

"Jazmean, I have to admit that I am having the time of my life and I don't want this night to end."

"It's not going to end anytime soon so let's enjoy it. Are you ready for dessert?"

"I'm ready for anything that you want to give me, baby."

"Well in that case, we can start with the pie I made for you."

"What kind is it?"

"It's your favorite, chocolate moose."
"You know me better than I thought."
"You should have known that, Shawn, after living with you I have gotten to know you more than I want to."
"There's still one thing you don't know about me."
"What is that?"
"How good I am in bed."
Jazmean hesitated to say anything because that was what she wanted to find out tonight. She looked into his eyes and said, "Tonight may be the night I find that out." Shawn surprised that she wanted him like that, just gave her a sexy smile and left the room.
"Where are you going, Shawn?"
"I'm going to get my chocolate moose pie so I can come back and eat it with you."
As Shawn left for the kitchen Jazmean took a deep breath. She was beginning to feel like she wasn't ready to sleep with Shawn, but now that she led him on she had to. To get her mind off that subject she began to clear the dishes off the table. As she headed for the kitchen Shawn was standing there.
"Where are you going so fast?"
"Just to put the dishes away. I'll be back."
"Don't be long. I already miss you."
Shawn stared at Jazmean from behind and started to think of what she looked like with *nothing* on. He shook his head and went to sit down so he wouldn't faint over Jazmean's beautiful body and the way she looked in that dress. Meanwhile, in the kitchen Jazmean was thinking about what Shawn looked like under his nice suit. She was imagining that she was touching his manly chest and his muscular arms. She couldn't help having chills running down her back. She blocked the image out of her mind and went out into the living room.
"Hey, baby, I'm back and I'm not going anywhere."
"In that case get your sexy self over here and eat some of this pie. It's beginning to look kinda good now that you're here."
Jazmean sat down beside him and started eating pie. Before long they were feeding each other and licking chocolate moose off of each other's fingers. They were almost finished eating the pie and they had enjoyed all of it.

"How do you like me now, Jazmean, I've shown you just how wild I can be."

"Yes, you did and I enjoyed watching you make a fool of yourself."

"Oh really, well how do you like this?" Shawn leaned over and kissed Jazmean on her lips as if to say 'you're mine and you're not getting away.' As he slowly pulled away after a long anticipated kiss, Jazmean was speechless. Her first impulse was to go for another kiss, but she didn't. She knew that if she did it would let him know that she wanted him like he wanted her. Instead she just played it cool.

"I liked that more than you know."

Shawn liked what he was hearing so he ran with it.

"So let's take it to another level." Jazmean wanted that so much, but she wanted him to suffer for a little while longer.

"You know that would be a dream come true, but first let's dance." Jazmean walked slowly over to put on some 'Hold Me' by 112 while Shawn was staring intently at her behind. As she walked back Shawn put his arms around her and they started to dance. He pulled her closer to him and let his hands slide down her back. Jazmean started to tense up as he got closer still to her butt. She tried not to show it by running her fingers across his neck to give him the same feeling of unlimited tension.

As they danced, things between them definitely were heating up. Instantly they both realized they wanted each other more and more by the minute. The music was still playing as they gazed passionately into each others eyes. At the heat of the moment, 'Anywhere' by 112 was playing. When Jazmean heard it she knew she couldn't keep it at this level for much longer. She moved closer to Shawn and kissed him with extreme desire. Shawn was ready for more.

He softly whispered, "You ready to experience the passion that I have for you?"

Jazmean didn't have to say a word. She pressed her thighs against his and ran her fingers erotically down the middle of his chest. Then she teased him with short, but smooth pecks of desire. She pulled away little by little from his lips and spoke softly, "Does that answer your question?"

That was all Shawn needed to begin his fulfillment of his yearning desire for her. Shortly they were undressing each other in the bedroom. It was going to be a night they wouldn't soon forget.

Chapter 3

It was morning and the sun shown through Jazmean's window. Shawn, still asleep, lay beside Jazmean with his arm across her chest. Jazmean was also asleep, curled up beside Shawn in a sense of security. The night had been one to remember. Full of emotion that had been held inside and was finally let out in one night of pure passion. It seemed for them like they couldn't resist each other any longer. All that happened in that one night could change their relationship for the better or the worse. They would soon find out it was really a mistake.

Buzz! Buzz! Buzz! The alarm clock was going off and neither of them seemed to hear it. They were in their own little world. Finally Shawn woke up and turned off the alarm.

"Jazmean, wake up baby you got to get ready for work."

Jazmean curled up closer to Shawn and said, "How would you like it if I just stayed here with you?"

"I would like it a lot, but you are so busy at the store you should go get caught up."

Jazmean smiled at Shawn as if to say she knew about all of that.

"Maybe, I can go in later and get caught up; that way we can continue what we started last night."

"It sounds like you want me to forget about my job, too."

"Well, if it comes to that, would you object?"

Shawn knew he wanted to stay there with her and reenact what they had done, but he just felt he had to get away for awhile.

"I'm sorry, baby, you know I want to stay here but I think I should go."

Beep! Beep! Beep! Beep!

Shawn reached over and grabbed his pager. The number was from Marco's house, and the message read: "9:00 Meeting." It was 7:30. This was a chance for Shawn to get away.

"Baby, you know I'm sorry. I have to meet my boss at the warehouse at 9:00, so I'm going to take a shower."

Jazmean looked at him with a sad face and said, "Well, I

guess you got to do what you got to do."

"I am truly sorry. Will you forgive me?"

"Just go, Shawn, I'll see you later."

Shawn got up and got in the shower. Jazmean began to pick up Shawn's clothes and put them away. She found the pants he had on the day before and felt something in the pocket. She pulled out a small bag of white powder. She knew *exactly* what it was and didn't know what to think. All that was going through her mind was, "Could Shawn be doing drugs? Is he that stupid to do drugs?" She was a combination of awestruck and sad at the same time. She could not believe that he, of all people, would have drugs especially some chronic cocaine. He knew better than that. She put it on the table and finished cleaning up.

"I'm going to kill him if he's using drugs," she said to herself. Shawn came out of the bathroom with a towel on.

"Shawn, we have to talk."

"About what? Did I do something wrong?"

"Yes. You could say it was wrong." Shawn looked confused. As he walked across the room he saw the drugs on the table and knew exactly what she wanted to talk about.

"Jazmean, let me explain." Shawn walked over to the table and picked up the cocaine and held it in his hand.

"So you admit that you're on drugs?"

"Jazmean, you know I wouldn't take drugs, but this *is* mine."

"Okay, if you're not taking drugs, what are you doing with it?"

"I wanted to tell you about this yesterday but we got all caught up. Look, I have this because it is part of my job."

Jazmean looked at him with the worst expression imaginable.

"You mean to tell me that your job is selling *drugs?*"

Shawn didn't think she would figure it out that fast. He couldn't even try to lie now; he had to tell her the truth.

"Yes, that's true. You have to let me tell you the whole story before you jump to conclusions."

"Fine, Shawn, go ahead; tell me your legitimate reason for having drugs in my house."

"First of all, I'm not saying that it's right, but I got a job as a runner for Marco. I only did it to make you happy and so you wouldn't have to worry about the bills."

"Shawn, I don't know what gave you the dumb idea that I would be happy with you selling drugs, but I'm not happy and *you* won't be happy once I finish this conversation. We don't need money so bad that you have to go work for the worst guy on the street. You and I both know that you can get a better job than that."

"If you want me to stop then I will, but this is just a quick way to make money."

Jazmean just looked at him. She didn't want to just say 'I hate you' and 'Get out I don't ever want to see you again.' She had only one thing on her mind, and that was to get him to realize he didn't need to sell drugs to make her happy.

"Shawn, I want you to stop working for Marco and get a real job. I don't want you to ruin your life and mine, too."

"I'll do anything for you, Jazmean, and you know that."

Shawn gave Jazmean a kiss on the cheek and said, "I've got to get dressed so I can go tell Marco I quit. I love you." He went to get dressed and left the apartment in silence.

Jazmean hoped that she had gotten through to Shawn. She didn't want to break up with him especially after she had had a wonderful time the night before. She loved him and she didn't want him to ruin his life when things were just getting good. She didn't want to give up *too soon*. Jazmean spent the rest of the morning wondering and worrying about Shawn.

Meanwhile, Shawn was on his way to meet Marco. All he could think of was what Jazmean said about him and the drugs. He knew he had to tell Marco he couldn't work for him anymore, but he wanted to live to see the next day. He knew how dangerous Marco was and what he could do. God would have to be on Shawn's side in order for him to get out of selling drugs for Marco. He had to give it a try for Jazmean and hope for the best.

"What's up, Marco, what's so important that you had to page me?"

Marco looked like he was ready to kill somebody and he

wasn't going to leave any witnesses. He stared right into Shawn's eyes and let him know it wasn't anything good.

"Well, Shawn, let me tell you that it is not a good thing."

"Tell me what it is then."

"I'll start by saying if you did it on purpose you better start apologizing now. The problem is that the merchandise that I gave you to give to my customer never got there. Now he is telling me he wants to get twice as much for the same price. As you should know, that messes up my business. What I want to know is did you deliver my merchandise to my customer."

Shawn froze. One way or the other he was going to get busted and he knew it. All he wanted to do was tell Marco he was quitting and leave. Now he had to come up with something to cover up his mistake.

Marco was getting impatient and said, "Well, are you going to answer my question?"

"Marco, I didn't deliver the merchandise because I forgot about it. I came here to give it back to you because I can't work for you anymore. I thought about it yesterday and I think that I should leave the running to one of your experienced workers. I just want to go find another job because I'm not good at this."

Marco listened to what Shawn had to say but wasn't taking it seriously.

"Listen, Shawn, I'm going to let you go ahead and quit because you haven't been here long, but if you ever come back wanting to work for me, I'm going to remember this."

Shawn was relieved that Marco didn't just go off and try to kill him, but he had a feeling that Marco had a catch. "What's the catch?"

"I'm glad you asked. I want you to do me a favor and get Jazmean's friend Shantell over here."

Shawn looked puzzled. What would a drug dealer like Marco want with Shantell? Was he going to try to get her to be his new *runner*?

"What do you want with Shantell?"

"I want her to take your place."

"What makes you think she would want to take my place?"

Marco paused for a minute. "Let me put it like this,

either you stay or she takes your place."

Shawn didn't want to drag Shantell, of all people, into this mess. All he wanted was a clean break. Marco was out to get something to benefit him. Shawn had to think of a way to quit working for Marco and keep Shantell out of harms way in the process.

"Can we leave Shantell out of this? She's Jazmean's friend and I don't want anything to happen to her."

Shawn was tense now. He hoped that Marco would come up with something else. Marco smirked a little and made it all seem like a joke.

"Well, there is one thing that could replace you besides her. I guess it would be three grand in cash by Thursday."

It was Monday. Shawn had seventy-two hours to get money. He figured it was better than giving up his girl's best friend.

"It's a deal. I'll have the money by Thursday night." Marco smiled satisfied with his agreement.

"Have it at Sr. Charles Pier at 8:30 p.m. sharp."

With that Shawn left without a word. Now he would have to come up with three grand out of nowhere. He knew the only way he could get it was ask his sister, LeAndra.

Chapter 4

LeAndra was Shawn's older sister. She owned a business and was making a lot of money. She always told Shawn that if he needed money he could come to her. Now was the time he needed her most. The only thing was that she was a *very* nosy sister and *always* wanted to know all of Shawn's business. Shawn rarely talked to his sister because of that and really hated that he would have to do it now.

Shawn drove over to LeAndra's house on the south side of town. All the way there he was trying to think of a reason for wanting to have so much money. He couldn't think of anything until he reached her house. At that moment it all came to him. He would tell her he was starting *his* own business.

"Hey, LeAndra, what's it like out here now days?"

"It's fine out here; it's no different from when you last came to see me three years ago."

"Has it been that long?"

"Yes, baby brother, it has."

"Well, I do apologize for that, but I'm here now."

LeAndra looked him in the eye as she always did to see if he was hiding something.

"Let me guess...you're here for some money."

He didn't say anything for a while but then he finally answered.

"Yes. I am here for money and I'm sure you have enough saved up to give me what I need."

LeAndra was not surprised. When he came to see her last time he asked for five hundred to pay his car payment. She was always nice enough to give it to him, but not without the usual question and answer session.

"How much do you need, when will I get it back, and what is it for?" Shawn really didn't want to answer all those questions but he did it just because he needed the money.

"I need three grand, you'll get it back by next year, and I need it to start my own business."

LeAndra didn't believe the last answer at all but she went along with it.

"So, what kind of business is it?"

"It's a...dance studio for...children."

He made it up off the top of his head and LeAndra knew it.

"That sounds good."

She didn't believe a word he said, but she walked over to her safe and took out the three grand.

"I think I will give you the money because of the children."

Now he was free. He had the money and now he just had to pay and get on with his life. Jazmean would be so happy for him if she knew what he had done. He wanted to tell her, but to be on the safe side he would keep it a secret.

"Thank you very much, LeAndra, I owe you a lot."

"It's seven thousand fifty-five dollars to be exact."

"I know, sis, I'll get it to you soon."

Shawn took the money and left. He now had 72 hours to clear his mind before confronting Marco again. He decided to go see Jazmean at work since he had free time.

"Hi, baby, how is your day going?"

Jazmean came from behind the counter and gave Shawn a big hug.

"My day is fine now that I see you. How is yours?"

Shawn didn't want to get into details so he just gave her a short story.

"Well, my day is fine now that I don't work for Marco anymore."

Jazmean was surprised. She didn't think that Shawn would get out of working for him that easy.

"What was the catch? What did he say you had to do for him?"

"Let's not talk about that. All that matters is that I can go get a good job now."

"It's about time you start using that degree in criminal justice you went to college for three years ago."

Shawn had forgotten all about that degree he worked so hard for.

"I wonder who would be hiring a criminal justice lawyer."

"A lot of people would hire a lawyer that is as good as you.

You should just go around to some firms and see what you can find."

"That's a great idea, baby, but I don't even remember how to write a résumé."

Jazmean covered her mouth to hide her laughter.

"How about I help you write your résumé and we go out together and find you a job."

Shawn was so happy Jazmean wanted to help him so much. He was really going to give it a try even though he was unsure of the out come.

"I think we can do that, Jazmean. You know I owe you one."

"Yes, I know you do but that can wait. Let's get started so you can help me around the apartment."

"I'll see you at home at around seven, right?"

"You know it."

Shawn left feeling surer of himself already. He was surer now than he had ever been. He would need that for what would happen next.

"Hello. Who is this?"

"This is your worst nightmare with a little surprise for you."

"Marco, I thought I told you my business with you was over. What is it that you have that would surprise me?"

"Well, Shawn, along with the three grand you're going to be giving me, I have decided to get my own little prize to go along with it."

Shawn was ready to think the worst. Knowing Marco he could have done anything to anyone and no one would be able to do anything about it.

"What 'little prize' did you decide to get?"

"I have your friend, Shantell."

"Marco! I thought we agreed to keep her out of this. What do you think this is a game?"

"Now calm down, Shawn, I haven't done anything yet."

"If you do **anything** you will have to except the consequences I have for you. Shantell means too much to me and Jazmean, and I will do anything to have you let her go."

Shawn was beginning to regret that he said that. Marco was good at coming up with things for people to do. He would have people do things you wouldn't imagine doing.

"Well, I actually have figured out something for you to do. It involves my money. I'm going to need you to bring it to me today."

"I can do that. Should I bring it to the same place?"

"Yes. The same time, too."

"I'll be there."

"Nice doing business with you."

"Whatever, Marco."

When Shawn hung up the phone he realized that Jazmean was coming home at seven. That meant he would have to make up something to be able to leave. He was sure that he would figure something out but he didn't know exactly what yet. The only good thing about giving Marco the money early was that he wouldn't have to worry about it anymore. It was 6:30 and he had thirty minutes to figure out something to tell Jazmean so he could leave. He was sure he would think of something.

Click. Click. Screech.

"I'm home, Shawn, where are you?"

"I'm in the kitchen come in here for a second."

"Did you miss me, baby?"

"You know I did, Jazmean that should be obvious."

Jazmean walked up behind him hugging his waist.

"So, what are we having for dinner?"

"If you keep sneaking up on me like that I'll be having *you* for dinner."

Jazmean quickly let go and rethought what Shawn had just said.

"Come on, Shawn, what are we *really* having for dinner?"

"Lasagna and bread sticks."

"Thank you. I'm going to change my clothes, and then we can eat."

Now was the time he needed to let her know that he would have to leave for awhile. He didn't know how she would take him telling her he was going to have to leave. He thought to himself, 'What do I have to lose?', so he went for it.

"Jazmean, could you come in here when you finish. I have something to tell you."

Jazmean walked into the kitchen while she was still trying to put on her shirt.

"What is it that you want to tell me?"

"I'm going to have to leave at around 8:00 because something came up with Marco."

"What is so important with Marco that would make you leave early on our night together?"

"Remember I told you that I didn't want to talk about not working for Marco anymore?"

Jazmean thought back. "Yes. What about it?"

Shawn hesitated.

"Well, I have to pay him three grand or he will do something to Shantell, or he will keep me working for him and have Shantell, too. That's why I have to leave."

Jazmean didn't know what to say. The fact that Shawn had gotten Shantell all mixed up in his drug game was the worse part. Jazmean would just have to let him go even though she didn't want to.

"Go! Just go and do what you need to do. I'm not hungry anymore."

"Jazmean, I don't want you to be mad at me. You know that if I could stay I would."

"Just go, Shawn!"

Shawn went to the bedroom, got the money, and left the apartment without a word. He thought to himself, 'I should have known she would take it this way. I should have told her what was going on from the beginning.' He hopped in his car and went speeding down Hilltop Drive. All he thought about was where he was supposed to be going...*Sr. Charles Pier 8:30*...that was all. It was only 7:30. He had an hour of free time, but it was supposed to be the time spent with Jazmean. Shawn was in over his head in all of his problems. He decided to go have a drink.

"What's up, Shawn? What can I get you today?"

"Ace, you can get me a cold beer."

"Well, then here you go."

Ace was Shawn's friend at the bar on 5th and Franklin. They had known each other since high school and they would do anything for each other.

"So, Shawn, what problems have sent you to a bar?"

"I got mixed up with Marco and now Jazmean is mad at me because I skipped out on our dinner plans for tonight."

"That was a big mistake. What was so important?"

"Like I told you I had gotten mixed up with Marco. I have to pay him his three thousand dollars or he will hurt Jazmean's friend, Shantell."

"Yo Shawn, you need to take a deep breathe and think for a minute about your situation. How long do you have to get the money to Marco?"

Shawn looked at his watch.

"I have exactly fifty-two minutes to get him his money. I just came here to take a deep breath like you said."

"So you *do* have the money."

"Yes, I do. Look, Ace, I need to get going because I really didn't want this to be question and answer time."

"All right, I'll catch you later."

Shawn left the bar and headed for the drop off spot. He was ready to get all this stuff with Marco squared away. Even if he was early it wouldn't hurt anybody.

"I pray to God this all works the way it's supposed to."

Chapter 5

Marco was driving up at 8:30 on the dot. Shawn was looking for Shantell but Marco hadn't brought her.

"Where is Shantell, Marco?"

Marco smirked and looked at Shawn.

"I don't believe she was part of the deal, my friend, she costs a little extra."

"I'm not a friend of yours and if Shantell is not part of the deal then we have no deal."

Shawn turned around and walked toward the car. He couldn't believe Marco would do something like that to him knowing that he would do anything for Shantell. Marco was getting really upset. He thought he could trust Shawn to come through for him.

"Shawn, I'm sure you can just give me the money and forget about the whole thing."

"You don't get it. I'm not going to just *forget* about my friend Shantell. If you did something to her you are going to pay with more than just three thousand dollars."

"Shantell was just something to get you to agree to give me the money early. I never even went to find her, so all you have to do is give me the money and this will all be over."

"So this is just a game to you? I don't trust you but here is the money. If I find out you did anything to her or you are lying I'm coming after you."

Shawn handed Marco the money and that was it. Shawn got in his car and headed for home, and Marco just disappeared.

"Jazmean, I'm back and I want to say I'm sorry."

"I'll be out in a minute."

Jazmean had been there by herself for two hours. In that time she started to feel weird so she took some medicine but that didn't help. She was in the bathroom when Shawn got there.

"I'll be in there in a minute, Shawn."

"Well, please hurry I want to talk to you."

Jazmean said to herself: 'I need to talk to you, too.' She walked out of the bathroom knowing Shawn was going to ask her what was wrong.

"What do you want to talk about?"

Shawn took a deep breath. He knew he just had to give it to her straight.

"Well, it's about Marco."

"Shawn. This is the last thing I want to hear tonight. You already walked out on me to complete the stupid deal with him, and now you have something else to tell me."

Shawn didn't expect that but he knew exactly how she felt.

"Listen, Jazmean, I gave Marco his money but I don't think he's going to leave it at that. I think he might try to mess with Shantell and try to get her involved in his little scams."

"Wait a minute; what does Shantell have to do with this whole mess with Marco anyway? She is my best friend and I don't want anything to happen to her."

Shawn was in too deep now. He was willing to just tell Jazmean the truth, but the odds were not in his favor.

"Marco told me before we made the money deal that he might exchange me for Shantell. But today he said he had Shantell with him and he would give her up for the money. The thing is that Shantell wasn't with him when I took him the money, but he told me he had never gotten her and was just saying that so he could get the money early."

Jazmean was full of questions about this whole thing. She started taking deep breaths to try to sort everything out.

"So you're telling me you think Shantell could be in some kind of danger with Marco?"

"Yes! I'm going to call her and make sure she is still all right, and then I will warn her about Marco."

"My head is still spinning from all of this. If you think it's best to check on her then you go ahead and do it."

Jazmean walked out of the room and left Shawn to call Shantell.

"Hello, this is Shantell."

"Shantell this is Shawn. I was just calling to check on you, and I need to tell you something really important."

"I'm fine. What is so important that you have to tell me at ten-thirty?"

"Well, I'm sure you know Marco, well he has made a threat to mess with you and get you caught up in his drug business. I'm calling to warn you that if you see him to get away as fast as you can."

"But, Shawn, what does Marco have to do with me? Why am I the one he's threatened to come after?"

Shawn took a long pause and was about to explain but realized it was pointless.

"Look, Shantell, it's a long story but I want you to take my advice."

"Okay, thanks but I've got to go."

Shawn hung up the phone and prayed Marco stayed away from Shantell. He was hoping that all of his worries were behind him. He wanted to get a new start on things. The number one thing in his life would be making Jazmean happy. He started to have second thoughts about it all. Was it *too soon* to just forget about all of it?

Shawn took a deep breath and walked back to the bedroom. Jazmean was sitting in a chair facing the window looking out at the view of Lake Michigan and the Chicago skyline. She was thinking about when she was a kid. Every day she would go running down by the lake to feed the birds. It was so peaceful back then. She wanted it to be the same way now, but time has changed everything. All in one day her dinner plans were ruined, she wasn't feeling good, and her boyfriend got her *best* friend caught up in all of his dirty business. She was wishing she could just start all over.

"Are you okay, Jazmean, you just walked away and didn't say anything."

Jazmean turned around and looked at Shawn with tears in her eyes.

"Shawn, some things are just bothering me right now and I don't know what to do."

"Come here, baby everything is going to be okay."

Shawn put his arms around her and gave her a kiss on her forehead.

"Whatever is wrong we can take care of it together okay, Jazmean. I'm not going anywhere."

Jazmean just relaxed in his arms and closed her eyes. She knew he would be right there for her no matter what.

"So are you going to tell me what's wrong or do I have to guess?"

"I don't feel too good right now and the medicine I took isn't working, plus you and all this stuff with Marco is driving me crazy."

"Jazmean, this thing with Marco should be over now so we don't have to worry about that, but let's go to sleep and see if you'll feel better in the morning."

Shawn swept her off her feet and laid her in the bed. Then he gave her a kiss and told her to close her eyes.

"Shawn, where are you going?"

"I'm going to turn off the lights and make sure the door is locked. I'll be right back just close your eyes and relax."

When he left the room he went and locked the door and turned off the lights. Then he paused for a minute and sat on the couch. He realized he was in so much trouble and that it was all because he had decided to get mixed up with Marco. He cleared his mind, went back to the bedroom, and fell asleep beside Jazmean.

Buzz! Buzz! Buzz! The alarm clock was going off but Shawn and Jazmean were still asleep so neither of them was going to move to turn it off. Finally Shawn woke up and turned it off. He lay back down and closed his eyes. Jazmean was still sleep and that's the way he left her. He got up and decided to make her breakfast. He had been a jerk and he needed to make it up to her. Twenty minutes later he had made eggs, bacon, waffles, and his special batch of orange juice. On top of all that he called Jazmean's job and told them she wouldn't be coming in.

He went into the bedroom and woke Jazmean up with a kiss.

"Wake up, Jazmean; I have a surprise for you."

"What kind of surprise do you have for me at seven in the morning?"

"Actually, its seven-thirty, but I can't tell you what the surprise is because then it wouldn't be a surprise."

Jazmean jumped up.

"Why didn't you wake me up? You know I have to go to work."

"The reason is that you're not going to work because I called in for you; plus you still have that surprise waiting for you. Now get up and come see your surprise."

Jazmean got up and started walking into the kitchen.

"You better have a good reason for keeping me home from work. You know I..."

She froze. She couldn't believe her eyes. Shawn had candles lit on the table and a wonderful breakfast for two.

"Speechless aren't you? Well, this is my way of apologizing for last night and all the other times I did something wrong. Is this a good reason for keeping you home?"

Jazmean didn't say anything. She just gave him a kiss and sat down at the table.

"Shawn, this is wonderful. I can't believe you took the time to do this for me."

"I needed to do it. By the way are you feeling better since you got some rest?"

"I'm feeling much better thanks to you. I just want to let you know that I'm not mad at you for last night. The only bad thing is that we didn't get to do your résumé."

"Let's forget about that until we finish our breakfast."

Shawn and Jazmean sat talking and eating the wonderful breakfast Shawn had made. Everything was beginning to look up for the two of them. Shawn was through with Marco and Jazmean was happy again. Things were going good, or *were they*.

Chapter 6

Three weeks had passed and things were going just perfectly. Jazmean had helped Shawn find a job that would express his qualifications at a Chicago law firm. He was getting paid good money and he was enjoying himself. Jazmean herself was having a great time at her job. She was happier now that Shawn was through with Marco. Shawn and Jazmean's relationship had improved. They were spending more time with each other and working out whatever problems they had. All was going well, or was it.....

Jazmean hadn't been feeling well for a little while now but she was just putting it out of her mind because she didn't think it was anything major. She thought it was normal.

Jazmean was working in her store that day and Shantell came in.

"What's up, Jazmean, you don't look so good."

"It's nothing I just haven't been feeling good for the past three weeks."

"You must be having some kind of problem because you haven't told me about your night with Shawn."

"I've just been busy since then and I have not had time."

"Well, are you going to tell me?"

"All you want to know is if I slept with him and I will tell you I did."

"You just go girl."

Shantell thought for a minute.

"Jazmean, you said you haven't been feeling good for three weeks and it has been three weeks ago when you slept with Shawn, so is it possible that you could be pregnant?"

Jazmean just froze. She had been sick since that night, she didn't use protection, and the odds were right for thinking that she was pregnant.

She cleared her throat and said, "It's possible, but I hope not."

"Well, that would explain why you've been sick for all this time. Go get one of those home tests and see if it comes out positive."

"Shantell, you know those things aren't 100% true. I

would have to go to a doctor to be completely sure."

"Then you do what you got to do. Don't put this off until tomorrow, do it tonight."

"Thank you for your advice, but I think I can handle this."

Shantell wanted to hear about every little detail and Jazmean knew that.

"Okay. I will tell you the results after I tell Shawn if I even do it."

Shantell just smirked at Jazmean. She knew Jazmean was stubborn.

"Okay, I guess I can wait until then. I will hope for the best for you and Shawn."

"You do that, Shantell, in the meantime I have to get back to work. I'll talk to you later."

Shantell left and Jazmean tried to put the whole situation in the back of her mind so that she could work. In spite of that she kept thinking of what Shawn would say when he found out. Would he freak out and leave her or would he stick by her no matter what? Jazmean's head was just full of unanswerable questions. She would just have to wait and see. She just couldn't keep stressing over all of this so she kept working.

Meanwhile, Shawn was hard at work. He was working on his first case and he was getting good at it. He was happier than ever because he had a real job and wasn't just hanging around the house doing nothing. He was very glad Jazmean had helped him get that job. All he could think about while he was at work was Jazmean. He had become so happy being with Jazmean. He had stopped going out with his 'boys' to the bars, and began to hang with Jazmean. Everything was cool, everything except with his friend, Andre.

Andre was Shawn's best friend. He hung out with him for a long time before he was with Jazmean. They told each other everything, but when Shawn got with Jazmean they lost a lot of their hang out time. Andre was coming to see Shawn at work to see how he was doing. This was the day Shawn had been waiting for.

Knock. Knock.

"Come in."

"What's up stranger?"

It was Andre. He loved to make surprise entrances.

"What's up, Andre, I haven't seen you in a long time either."

"Well, you know how work gets, I've just been caught up and I haven't been able to get away."

"So, what is your excuse?"

Shawn didn't want to mention his former business with Marco, so the next best excuse would be Jazmean."

"You know how it is. Jazmean and I have been kind of busy together these past few weeks and I have just started this new job. Things have cut off my free time."

"All right, I understand I have kind of been talking to a female myself. She has kept me busy, too."

Shawn looked at Andre in surprise. Andre had never let a female keep him busy.

"Who is the lucky woman that can keep *you* busy?"

Andre cleared his throat trying not to be embarrassed.

"Her name is Crystal and she is worth my time. She is a professional singer and when she's in town she wants me to herself."

"Well, I'm happy for you and Crystal. What do you say we go get something to eat and catch up on lost time?"

"I wish I could but I'm going to met Crystal for lunch. I will catch up with you later and take you up on that offer."

Shawn was glad that Andre found him someone but he was kind of disappointed he didn't have time to grab a bite to eat.

"Good luck to you and Crystal and I'll catch you later."

Andre left and Shawn sat back down in his big chair to work and decided to skip lunch. He had a lot to do anyway.

Meanwhile, over at World Read bookstore, Jazmean was still pondering the thought of being pregnant. While she was still in her daze, her sister Teresa walked in. She was looking for an Italian cookbook. When Jazmean saw her she had a feeling she was up to something.

"Teresa, what brings you here to my store?"

"I came looking for an Italian cookbook."

"Who are you cooking Italian for?"

"I'm cooking it for Tyrek because he needs something new

in his diet."

Jazmean laughed.

"You know Tyrek doesn't eat anything but his mom's old cooking."

Teresa got offended by that and snapped at Jazmean.

"How can you tell me anything about my man when your so-called man has no job and doesn't care what he eats?"

"Look, Teresa, Shawn is a person just like Tyrek."

"Well, while we're on your man, does he have a job yet? Does he bring home some good money or do you do everything?"

Jazmean tried to hold back but she just went for it anyway.

"Let me tell you something. Shawn has a good job as a lawyer and he is better to me then Tyrek could ever be to you."

Teresa was tongue tied. She didn't have anything else bad to say about Shawn.

"I'm sorry! Can I just pay for my book and go?"

Jazmean took Teresa's money and Teresa left without another word. That argument about Shawn made her think more about what he would do if she was pregnant. She felt she just *had* to call Shawn so she did.

"Hello. This is Shawn. Can I help you?"

"It would help if you were here with me."

Shawn knew it was Jazmean and he was happy to talk to her.

"Hey, baby, I really wish I could be there, but I am pretty busy."

"Well, what time do you get off work?"

"I get off at six-thirty, how about you?"

"I get off at five, so I'll be home before you."

Shawn was kind of disappointed but he knew she would be okay with it.

"Well, I should get back to work so that I can leave on time. I love you."

"Much love to you, too, Shawn. I'll see you when you get home."

They both hung up the phone happier then when the got on. Jazmean was just thinking about the time she would be home before Shawn came home. She would use that time to find out the results of the test. For now she needed to work.

It was 3 hours later and Jazmean was closing up the store. All the other employees were gone and she was there by herself. When she left the store she headed for the corner drug store. She quickly went in and bought her pregnancy test, not believing she was really buying the test, and then left as quickly as she came.

When she got home she checked her messages. There was one from Shawn saying he would be home a little after 6:30 so don't wait up. Jazmean was happy that she had some more time to think of how to tell Shawn after she had the results. She couldn't wait any longer to try to prove Shantell wrong so she went to take the test. Fifteen minutes later she had the answer. Shantell was right. Jazmean was pregnant. Now she had to let Shawn know about it. The time pasted really fast and that moment was there sooner than she expected.

Shawn came into the room in the greatest mood, but when he saw that Jazmean wasn't too happy his mood changed.

"What's wrong, Jazmean."

"I just have something to tell you, but I don't know how you're going to take it."

"Well, you won't know until you tell me."

Jazmean took a deep breath. This was the moment of truth.

"You know how I haven't been feeling good for the past few weeks?"

"Yes, Jazmean, I know about it."

"Well, I found out why that is."

"Are you going to tell me or do I have to guess?"

"It's because I'm...pregnant."

Shawn couldn't say anything. So many thoughts were going through his mind.

"Are you telling me I'm going to be a father? Why does this have to happen now?"

"I feel the same way but we have to deal with it."

"*We?* I'm not ready to deal with a child. I just got myself together what can I do for a child?"

"Shawn, I'm not ready for a baby either, but I'm having

one."

"Well, you didn't talk to me about children so soon so what can I do?"

"For now you can support me."

Shawn didn't want to hear that cause all of this was hitting him so hard he just couldn't take it. He stormed out of the apartment without another word. He got in his car and sped away. As he drove he was thinking about what he was going to do about this child that they would be having. He really wanted to put it out of his mind so he headed for the bar on 5th and Franklin.

"What can I get for you, Shawn?"

"Just give me a straight gin with a lemon twist."

"Whoa, man, what's got you drinking like this?"

Shawn gave Ace a look of disgust.

"Jazmean just told me that she is pregnant and I just don't know what I'm going to do about it."

Ace was shocked and amazed at this news.

"Well, I want to say congratulations but you might bite my head off. If I were you I wouldn't be in a bar drinking, I would be at home with my girlfriend."

Shawn was getting upset because Ace was giving him advice he didn't want.

"Look, Ace, I'm not you and I don't want your advice. I'm not ready for a baby."

"I'm sorry man I just want to help."

"You can help by giving me another drink."

Ace wasn't going to give Shawn another drink and then let him go drive on the road. If he was going to help him he had to keep him from drinking anymore.

"I'm sorry, Shawn, but I can't give you anymore if you're going to be driving home."

Shawn thought about it and Ace was right.

"I need to go anyway. I'll see you around."

Shawn left the bar and just drove. The next thing that popped into his mind was: 'What would mom think if she found out Jazmean was pregnant.' He couldn't let her find out from someone else so he headed over to her house. When he pulled up into the driveway his mom was coming out the door to ask him why he was there.

"What is it now, Shawn, are you in some kind of trouble or something?"

"Can I get out of the car first before you start grilling me for answers?"

Shawn's mom, Brenda, liked to get answers from her children. Ever since Shawn was little, Brenda would ask him questions about everything.

"Come on in, Shawn, but you're going to answer my questions."

"Okay, mom, will do."

Shawn turned off the car and went up to the front porch. When he got in the door she was back with more questions.

"So, why are you here? Are you in some trouble?"

Shawn took a deep breath to get ready to answer all of his mom's questions.

"I just wanted to come see you and I wanted to tell you something."

"Now you know you didn't just come to see me. You would rather be over there with Jazmean then out here with me."

"Not today, mom, Jazmean just told me something that I wasn't ready to hear."

"What did she tell you?"

"She told me she was pregnant."

Brenda was surprised but she wasn't upset.

"Well, what are you going to do about it?"

"I don't know. I'm not ready for this."

"The least you can do is support her and be there with her."

"I just wanted to know from you if you were upset about this."

"No, why should I be? I will have my first grandchild. You know your sister doesn't want any kids. By the way does LeAndra know?"

"No. She doesn't know and I want to keep it that way."

"Fine. She won't hear it from me. You should go and be with Jazmean now and let her know how you feel."

Shawn thought about it and realized that he had just run

out on her.

"Thanks, mom, I think I will do that."

Shawn got in his car and headed for home. He was thinking about what he would say to her when he got there.

Chapter 7

As Shawn pulled up in the parking lot he was thinking of Jazmean. As he walked up to the door, he thought of how happy she made him. Shawn unlocked the door and went in. Jazmean was sitting on the couch crying. Shawn felt worse at that moment than he had ever felt before.

"Jaz, I want to say I'm sorry for walking out on you like that. I should have been here supporting you."

Jazmean didn't say, or do anything she just sat there.

"Look, Jazmean, I know I was wrong but the least you can do is talk to me."

"Shawn, what you did was so wrong! You made me think you didn't care about me anymore."

Shawn had to let her know he cared. He walked over to her and held her in his arms.

"Baby, I don't care what happens I'm not going to stop caring about you. What we need to do right now is get a good night's sleep so we can talk about this in the morning."

Jazmean surrendered to Shawn and went with him into the bedroom. She fell asleep in Shawn's arms and he held her all night. He made a promise to himself that he would never leave her like that again.

It was morning and Shawn and Jazmean still lay peacefully in their bed. They had a busy day to look forward to. Shawn would have another case to do and Jazmean would have more books to sell. After the night before, things were going back to normal really quickly. Even though they still had a lot to talk about, they would still go back to their normal life. They really didn't have a choice.

"Jazmean, wake up, it's time for you to get ready for work."

Jazmean didn't really want to go to work, but she didn't want to let Shawn know that.

"Okay, fine. I'm getting up."

Jazmean got up and left the room. After she had left the room the phone rang.

"Hello."

"Hey, this is Shantell. Is Jazmean there?"

"Yeah, she's here but she's getting ready to go to work. What do you want me to tell her?"

"Tell her that I'm coming by the store to talk to her."

"I'll do that."

"Thanks."

After Shawn got off the phone Jazmean came back into the room to get something.

"Shantell just called and told me to tell you that she's coming to the store to talk to you."

"Okay thanks, Shawn. Oh, I wanted to let you know that I won't be coming home right after work today."

Shawn was puzzled. Why wouldn't she come home?

"Where are you going after work?"

"To see a doctor to make sure I'm okay. There's nothing to worry about."

"You know we have to talk about this baby thing when you get home."

Jazmean was surprised that Shawn actually cared enough to want to talk about it.

"It's a deal. I'll be home before you know it. Now go get ready for work or you'll be late."

Jazmean hurried out the door and Shawn went to get dressed for work. Even though the two of them hadn't done much talking, Shawn felt like Jazmean was taking this pregnancy thing pretty well. He, on the other hand, was not sure if he could make it through having a child of his own. In the end of all of his doubtfulness he was ready for the challenge. The first thing he had to do was go to work.

Meanwhile, Shantell was sitting at home and the phone rang.

"Hello. This is Shantell."

"Hello. This is your dream come true."

"Who are you? Is this a joke?"

"No it's not a joke. This is Jose the one you met at "Hotties in Hizhouse". I am finally calling you because I want to take you up on your offer."

Shantell was trying to think of what offer he was talking about. It had been three weeks and she hadn't even thought about Jose.

"What offer are you talking about, Jose?"

"The offer you gave me on the card. You said that if I need a friend to call you, so that's what I'm doing."

Shantell remembered the card now but she realized that it was 8:30 in the morning.

"I don't mean to let you down but I don't need to be talking to you at 8:30 in the morning about being your friend. Maybe if you call around noon we can talk."

Jose didn't really realize that he had called her so early. It was a spare of the moment thing to call her.

"I am sorry about calling you so early but I do want to get to know you."

"That's fine and all but it is early."

"I respect that, so I'll call you later."

Jose had hung up and Shantell started to laugh at the fact that Jose had called so early in the morning. Then she remembered why she had woken up so early in the first place. She was going to get the scoop on Jazmean. She didn't wait any longer to rush over to Jazmean's store. She grabbed her keys and was out the door.

When she got to the store it seemed like Jazmean was waiting for her.

"I'm glad your here, Shantell, now you can grill me on what happened with Shawn even though I don't want to tell you."

"Very funny, Jazmean, I've had enough of your jokes. Tell me what happened."

"Well, first of all I am pregnant and second when I told Shawn he got really quiet then he turned into a monster, told me he wasn't ready for a baby, and stormed out of the house to go who knows where."

"Did he come back? Was he still mad?"

"Yes, he came back but he wasn't mad. He was really calm and apologized for leaving me like that. Then since I was so upset he held me in his arms as I fell asleep."

Shantell didn't think it would turn out like this. She figured he would leave and not come back, or they would still be fighting about the situation.

"So is he cool with the baby thing?"

"You know what, I don't know. This morning he said that we needed to talk after I got home. I don't know what he's going to say. Anyway, enough about me, you've been kind of not telling me about your life for awhile."

"Well, the only thing that has happened to me lately is that this guy I met at the club named Jose called me at 8:30 this morning."

"What for?"

"He said he was calling to take me up on my offer to be his friend. Since it was early in the morning I told him to call later and we would talk."

Jazmean wanted to laugh because of the fact that this guy would call her so early in the morning. She held it in and listened to Shantell.

"He must really be interested in you to have the nerve to call you at 8:30."

"Whatever you say, I've got to go so I'll talk to you later."

"All right I'll talk to you later about your new *boyfriend.*"

Jazmean continued working and laughing about what happened to Shantell. She was glad someone was able to make her laugh and forget a little bit about the situation she was in. She just hoped Shawn was getting through his day. She knew he was kind of not sure about what to do about her being pregnant. No matter what, she would *still* love him.

All the while, Shawn was at work. He was still thinking about that morning and the day before, but he wasn't mad about it anymore. He had realized he had another responsibility now and he had to face it like the others. Since he would need more money, he would have to hold out on paying his sister back the seven thousand fifty-five dollars he owed her. He had collected the three thousand all ready, but now he needed to keep it. He thought he was off the hook a little *too soon.*

Chapter 8

When five o'clock came Jazmean was out the door and on her way to see a doctor. She had confidence that everything was all right and she wouldn't have anything to worry about. It was true. The doctor said she was just fine and all she needed to do was eat healthy and remember that she had a baby inside her. After that she was happy and surer that everything would workout. When she got home Shawn was waiting for her.

"So how did it go?"

Shawn was anxious to find out if Jazmean and the baby were okay.

"It went fine, Shawn. The doctor said all I really need to do is remember to eat healthy and take care of myself."

Shawn was relieved to hear good news and not bad.

"That's good. I want to let you know that I want to be here with you and help you out when you need it."

"That's kind of surprising coming from a guy who four weeks ago didn't have a job and wouldn't even help clean up the house."

Shawn was shocked. What gave her the nerve to say that? Shawn didn't know but he was about to find out.

"What is that suppose to mean? Does it mean you think that I'm not capable of helping anyone? Does it mean I just want to have people do things for me and not do *something* for them?"

"Shawn, you don't have to get an attitude. I didn't mean it like that at all."

Shawn didn't even know why he was getting so upset.

"I'm sorry, Jaz, it's just that I'm trying so hard to meet your standards. I guess I'm trying *too* hard."

"It's okay you don't have to worry so much anymore. We're going to be fine."

Shawn wanted so much to make everything right and have Jazmean believe that he wanted to help and that she could trust him. When she went back to the old idea about him not having a job or helping her, he went off the deep end. That was the last thing he wanted to hear after all that had happened. He was trying to make a new life for the both of them, but Jazmean's comment just set him back a step. He didn't worry about it though because he was still going to move forward.

"So when are you going to tell your family about this?"

Jazmean hadn't thought about that yet. She was barely getting the information herself.

"Have *you* told any of your family yet?"

"Yeah. While I was out yesterday I went to see my mom. I talked about it with her and she's cool with it. The only thing is that I haven't told LeAndra about it."

"Are you going to?"

"Yes."

"Well, I was going to call my mom, but maybe I should go see her."

"That's cool with me. I don't have anything planned for us so you can go now if you want."

"I think I'll do that."

Jazmean left on her way to her mother's house to tell her the news.

Shawn left soon after that to go break the news to his sister. Even though he had said he wasn't going to tell her he felt that he should. Besides that, she would be upset if she found out from someone else that Shawn is going to have a child and can't pay her the money he owes her. It would be best if she heard it from him.

Knock. Knock. Knock.

"It's about time... oh it's just you."

"Is that anyway to greet your brother?"

"I'm sorry, Shawn, I was just expecting someone else. What are you here for anyway?"

Shawn was just waiting for her to ask him that.

"I came to let you know something before you find out from someone else."

"Is it about what you *really* did with the money I gave you?"

Shawn smiled and said, "No it's not about that, but it does have something to do with the money. I'm not going to be able to pay you back as soon as I told you I could, because something has come up."

LeAndra rolled her eyes like she knew he was going to say

that.

"What came up, Shawn?"

"That's what I came to tell you; Jazmean is pregnant."

LeAndra's mouth dropped. She forgot all about the money for a minute and was happy for Shawn and Jazmean.

"I don't know what to say. I never thought you would have a kid before I did. I'm happy for you little brother."

Shawn was kind of surprised because he didn't think she would take it that easily. He was ready for her to be mad about not getting her money. Instead she was happy for him and didn't care about the money.

"I'm glad you're not upset, but I didn't expect you to be this happy."

"You really think I would be upset over some money? You can give me back the money later, but right now you have a higher priority to deal with than money. You're going to be a father, and that's more important then a few thousand dollars. Besides there's more money were that came from."

"So everything is cool then, right?"

"Yeah, little brother, everything is cool as long as you take good care of my little niece or nephew, and take care of Jazmean."

"I don't have a problem with that."

Shawn and LeAndra continued to talk about Jazmean and the baby. They were getting along pretty well considering Shawn barely talked to his sister before all of this happened. Their conversation was going well until LeAndra started to be a little more curious about the situation.

"Shawn, I have a question for you that you probably won't want to answer, but I'm going to ask anyway."

Shawn got kind of suspicious about that. His sister was good at turning a good conversation into a bad one.

"What do you want to ask?"

"It's about you and Jazmean. Are you going to..."

"Hold it right there, LeAndra, I don't know if I want to hear this."

"Oh chill out, Shawn, it's going to come up anyway."

"Fine go ahead."

"Are you going to marry her?"

Shawn was dead silent after that. What could he say to that question? He hadn't even thought about talking about marriage with Jazmean, let alone asking her to marry him. LeAndra did have a point though. Jazmean would have a link to him from now on and there was nothing he could do about it.

"LeAndra, you really caught me off guard with that one. I haven't even thought about that. You know what, Jazmean and I will always be linked together by that baby from now on so it's not out of the question. I just need some time to think about it."

"You do all the thinking you want. I can tell you one thing, I am happy with my husband even though he's not here most of the time. All I want to say is it wouldn't be a bad idea, but you should think about it for a while before you decide."

"Thanks, sis, you can always bounce me back into shape after you stretch me out. I will think about it and eventually talk about it with Jazmean."

"Good. That's all I want you to do."

"Well I should go now. I have some work to do before Jazmean gets home."

"Okay I'll see you."

Shawn left and went home. He was thinking about the marriage thing pretty hard. He didn't want to let Jazmean go and he wasn't even interested in anyone else, so he wouldn't be losing anything. Then again he didn't want to scare Jazmean off with a marriage proposal. He would just have to think a little bit more.

Meanwhile, Jazmean was at her mother, Marisa's house. She had been there for a little while when her sister Teresa came over. Teresa was just coming to see her mother since she hadn't in awhile. They had begun a conversation about each other, but the baby situation hadn't come up yet. Just then Jazmean's father Andrew came in from work. Jazmean thought it would be as good a time as any to bring the situation up.

"Mom, Dad, Teresa, there is something I want to talk to you about."

She got her father's attention and he was all ears.

"What is it, baby girl? You can tell daddy."

"Well, dad you know I have been seeing Shawn for 5 months now and we are getting really close, and..."

Teresa butted in and put her two cents in.

"You know, dad, Shawn is not really good for Jazmean. You should make her let him go."

"Teresa, stop butting in. I want to hear what my daughter has to say. Go ahead Jaz."

"First of all there is no chance now that I am going to leave Shawn. Now as I was saying we are together and there is no easy way to say what I'm going to say."

Marisa was getting impatient.

"Just go ahead and say it. It can't be that bad."

"I am.....pregnant by Shawn."

Complete silence filled the room. Marisa couldn't do anything but sit there. Andrew just had a puzzled look on his face. Teresa couldn't believe she hadn't told her when she talked to her last time.

"Well, somebody has to say something before I start to think you want to kill me."

"Trust me, we don't want to kill you," Marisa said, "When did you find out about this?"

"I found out a couple of days ago."

Teresa said, "Does Shawn know?"

"Yes he knows. He was the first one I told."

Andrew was just pacing back and forth during all of this. He hadn't said a word since she announced the pregnancy.

"Daddy, are you going to say something?"

"Jazmean, what happened to all the stuff we taught you? Did it just fly out of the window?! You should know that I'm not too happy with this."

"Shawn and I are working and everything is going to be fine."

"Have you forgotten that I wanted you married before you had kids? Besides that you are the baby girl. Your brother and sister don't have any kids."

"Dad! You can't compare me to them. Frederick is in prison and I don't care what Teresa does. They are not even like me. I can handle whatever situation I am in with or without your help."

"Jazmean don't raise your voice to your father."

"What! Mom, do you agree with him?"

"No. I believe in you, and I trust you to do what you need to do. I am happy for you."

"Okay fine, you can say your happy now when the baby is not here, but I am here to tell you I am having my baby, and I don't care what you think. I just thought you all should know."

Andrew was even madder now.

"You need to care about what we think! You are still my child and I still love you. I want to know why you want to mess up your life with a baby. You're not even married yet!"

"The truth is I haven't even thought of marriage, but if he were to ask me, I would say yes. I love Shawn and there is nothing you can do about that. I didn't plan for this baby, no, but I still know what I have to do. I am twenty-four years old and soon I will be twenty-five. You have to stop treating me like I am fifteen."

"All right, maybe I am worrying too much and treating you like a fifteen year-old, but you know why."

"Look, I have had enough of this. If I need to talk to you I'll call first."

Jazmean left not really knowing what her parents and sister *really* thought about her having a baby. The truth was that by now she didn't care what anyone thought about her, or her baby, all she wanted was for Shawn to love her, and be by her side. Nothing could stop her now only because she was determined to make it.

It was 9:00 when Jazmean got home. She was tired and she knew she just needed to get some rest, so she just put everything down and went into the bedroom. Shawn was already in a deep sleep so Jazmean just lay down beside him and went to sleep.

Chapter 9

Beep! Beep! Beep! Beep! Buuzzzzzz! Buuzzzzz! It was morning, Shawn's pager was going off, and so was the alarm clock. Jazmean jumped up to turn off the alarm clock, and Shawn jumped up to turn off his pager. When everything was quite again Jazmean and Shawn looked at each other and lay back down on the bed.

"So, Jaz, what time did you come back last night?"
Jazmean yawned and looked at Shawn.
"I got here at nine and I didn't want to wake you."
"You could have just to let me know you were home."
"Who just paged you?"
"Oh, that was my boss reminding me of the meeting at eight. Don't worry I will get there."
"It really doesn't matter to me after the night I had."
"I meant to ask you how it went with your mom."
"I had more then just my mom to deal with. My dad and sister were there, too."
"How did they take it?"
"I'm not really sure about my mom and Teresa, but dad didn't take it well at all."
Shawn knew that would be her father's reaction, but he was hoping that it would be different.
"I'll bet he was madder at me then he was at you."
"I guess you can say that, but it doesn't bother me. He's just my father he can't really do anything. Let's just forget about him and have a good day, okay."
Jazmean got up and left the room. Jazmean was right; they didn't need to worry about her dad. They would make it and Shawn knew it.
Shawn got up, got his clothes together, and waited for Jazmean to finish getting dressed. When Jazmean came back into the room Shawn gave her a kiss and went to take a shower. By the time Shawn got finished Jazmean had already left. Shawn headed out of the door to go to his meeting.

Meanwhile, Shantell was heading out of the door to go to

her job. Right when she was about to leave the phone rang.
"Hello?"
"Hello, this is Jose."
"Jose, I *really* want to talk to you, but I'm kind of headed out of the door to go to work."
"Where do you work?"
"Macy's on 12th and Grand. Look, I really have to go."
"I'll be coming by to see you so don't leave early."
"Okay, bye."

Shantell hung up the phone and left for work thinking about Jose.

Over the past few days Shantell and Jose had become close and they were getting to know each other. Shantell was beginning to think that Jose was the one for her. Jose was thinking all of it was just too good to be true. Together they were just two confused people. They liked it that way.

At World Read, Jazmean was working away. She was having more customers then usual because she got a new book in. Even though she was busy she was still thinking about Shawn. In the middle of her thoughts Teresa walked in.

"Well, isn't this a surprise? Did you come to bite my head off like dad did yesterday?"

Teresa looked at Jazmean innocently.

"No, this time I came just to buy a book. Is 'Acts of Taylor' in yet?"

"It's over in the corner."

Jazmean laughed as Teresa walked back to get her book. Jazmean really thought that she had come just to grill her on the baby thing.

"Okay, I'm ready to buy it now. One more thing, are you really taking what dad said seriously?"

"No, I'm not. Dad is just being a dad and he can't help but be over protective. I'm his little girl."

"I'm glad because what he said was kind of harsh. Anyway, that's not what I'm here for. How much does this book cost?"

Jazmean laughed a little.
"Eight dollars."

Teresa paid for her book and left. Jazmean continued

working like nothing had happened. Just then Shantell walked in.

"What's up, girl, I only came for a few minutes to say hi."

"How are you today? Are you headed for work?"

"Yes. I almost couldn't get out of the door because Jose called me."

"What's up with you and him lately?"

"Oh, there's a little "something, something" go on between us but it's pretty much just friendly stuff."

"Next thing you know he's going to want to come to your house and spend the night."

Shantell smirked and rolled her eyes. She knew Jazmean was headed for that angle of things.

"It's not like that at all. Well, I've got to go now so I will call you later."

Shantell rushed out and Jazmean just shook her head and grinned.

"Shawn, I'm glad you could make it. This is a very important meeting. We have a new client and he is not known as a good boy out on the street, but we are going to treat him like anyone else we would represent."

"Who is this new client?"

"His name is Marco Kendricks and he is in trouble with a few bad cops. He's looking at fifteen years unless we help him."

Shawn just dropped his head. A few weeks ago Marco was out of his life and now he would be a client he might have to work with.

"Well, who is he assigned to?"

"I have thought about that and I picked you."

"I'm sorry, sir, but I don't think I would be the best to represent him."

"Why is that?"

"I have some past issues that I had with him and I just don't want to get involved in his case."

Shawn's boss took a minute to think about it and came up with his answer.

"I'm sorry about whatever happened in the past, but you are the only one that is free and has only one case. I hope you can put behind you the hard times and just do your job. Are you going to have a problem with that?"

Shawn really didn't want the case but he sucked all of his hate for Marco in and thought about taking the case.

"No, I'm not going to have a problem with it."

"Good. He will be coming in at two o'clock to meet with you."

"Thank you."

Shawn got up and left the meeting knowing that something bad was going to come out of him representing Mr. Kendricks.

While he was in his office he started looking at Marco's file and seeing what he could do to help his already weak case. He was beginning to think it would be hopeless to defend Marco. He already didn't like him. It didn't make it any better when two o'clock hit and Marco was on his way to Shawn's office.

"Hello, Mr. Kendricks, come in and have a seat."

Marco looked at Shawn with a devious look on his face.

"Are you my lawyer?"

"Yes, I am. Now have a seat so we can get started."

Marco knew that Shawn was kind of uncomfortable with being his lawyer, so he decided to make a little comment.

"It's pretty nice that after you worked for me you managed to get a job like this."

"Look, Marco, I don't have time to play your little games. I'm here to be your lawyer and that's it. Now tell me your side of the story."

After that speech Marco gave up trying to be sarcastic anymore. He just did what Shawn asked him to do because he knew he needed a lawyer and Shawn would just have to do.

After Marco left Shawn was ready to go home. Marco had just about gotten on Shawn's last nerve. Shawn was just so tired of the way Marco was acting.

After a while Andre came to see Shawn.

"What's up, Shawn, how's your day going?"

Shawn looked up and saw Andre and was glad it wasn't Marco.

"My day has been horrible until now, how about yours."

"My day is good compared to yours. I came by to see if you

wanted to go to lunch."

Shawn sighed. He had so much work to do but he really wanted to kick it with Andre.

"You know what, I wish I could go to lunch with you but I am so busy. I have a new case to work on."

"No problem, I could come to dinner one day."

"That would be a great idea. Maybe you can bring your new girlfriend with you and finally get to see Jazmean."

"So, what's up with you and Jazmean, anyway?"

Shawn smiled like he was proud of being with Jazmean.

"We are having a baby and I'm pretty happy about that."

Andre was shocked. His boy would be a father before him.

"Yeah that is cool. I am happy for you, man. I wish you the best of luck."

"I'm happy, too."

"Well, you know what, I've got to go. I'll talk to you later."

Andre left and Shawn sat down to do his work.

Meanwhile, Shantell was at Macy's working hard doing her job. She still was thinking about Jose. The next thing she knew Jose was standing in the door with a dozen roses in his hand. He was dressed in a black suit and a blue shirt and tie. Shantell's eyes nearly popped out of her head. As Jose walked over to her she was anticipating what he was going to say.

"Hello, sweet thing, I told you I would be coming to see you."

Shantell was nearly speechless at the fact that Jose looked so good and sounded so sexy.

"I...uh...don't know what to say. You look as fine as a bottle of wine in that suit."

Jose grinned and replied to her daring response.

"Wait until you see what I look like without this suit on."

Shantell nearly lost her breath after that.

"Hold up, let's not go that far. We are just getting to know each other. What are you here for anyway besides surprising me with a dozen roses?"

"I came to ask you to lunch with your fine self."

"Where are we going?"

"I'm going to the Italian restaurant down the street. Is that fine with you?"

"Yes, let's go."

Jose grabbed Shantell's hand and they laughed out of the store on their way to lunch.

It seemed as though everything was going great for everyone and nothing could go wrong. Jazmean and Shawn were happy. Shantell and Jose were getting together and becoming close friends. Teresa and Jazmean's family was excepting the fact that Jazmean was pregnant. LeAndra cancelled all of Shawn's debt because of the baby. Every worry that was bothering them was disappearing. It was a good thing because what would happen next would make things all together *worse*. Things were about to get *ugly*.

Chapter 10

It was three weeks later, everything was going just fine. Shawn had the big trial with Marco coming up that day and he was afraid he would lose. Jazmean tried to cheer him up and let him know that even if he lost it would be okay. What she didn't know was whom he had the case with. She was about to find out.

"So who are you defending?"

Shawn looked at Jazmean.

"I don't want you to get scared because I have it under control. I am defending Marco Kendricks."

"You mean to tell me that you are defending the man that almost ruined your life?"

"Yes. I have no choice."

"The hell you don't. You should have told your boss you didn't want his case."

"Jaz, I told the boss I had bad history with Marco, but he said I needed to put it behind me and just do my job."

"All I have to say is that you better watch your back. If you lose God knows what he might do."

"I wish I could change things, but the trial is today so just wish me luck."

Shawn got his things and walked out the door.

"What the hell is wrong with him?", Jazmean thought to herself.

He was right in a way; all she could do was wish him luck. She had other things like work to think about. Shawn would just have to go through the trial with faith in God.

Riinngg! Riinngg!

"Hello."

"Tell your man I will be waiting for him."

After that the phone clicked and there was nothing else. Jazmean knew it had to be Marco. Now she was even more scared then before, but what could she do. She couldn't take being in the house any longer so she went off to work.

When she got there Shantell was waiting for her.

"How's it going, Jazmean?"

"I hope you are here to take my mind off of Shawn because if you're not you can leave."

"Wait just a minute. What's up with you and Shawn?"

"Shawn has to defend Marco Kendricks in court today and there is nothing I can do about it."

"Why would he choose to do that?"

"His boss made him put his past with Marco behind him so he could do his job. I don't like it one bit, and besides Marco called this morning talking about tell your man I will be waiting for him."

"That's kind of deep. I hope Shawn realizes what he's gotten into."

"I do, too."

"I didn't come to take your mind off of Shawn, even though it would help. I came to tell you about Jose."

"You're still talking to Jose?"

"Yes."

"Are you two serious?"

"You could say that. For the last three weeks he has come to my job every other day to bring me candy or flowers. If that's not serious I don't know what is."

"It sounds serious to me. So what's up between the two of you?"

"Just the same old stuff; I have to say that he is a perfect gentleman."

"Has he asked to spend the night at your house yet?"

Shantell laughed and looked at her with a joking face.

"No he hasn't, but he has made little remarks in that direction. I think he will wait until I am ready before he goes that far."

"That's a good thing. You know I should get to work now. I will call you later."

"Talk to you then."

Shantell left and Jazmean was happy again.

Things weren't so great at Shawn's office. He had lost Marco's file then when he finally found it in his briefcase it wasn't finished. He had to work extra hard to get it finished before they went to court. It wasn't any better when Marco himself came into Shawn's office.

"Are you ready to win me this case?"

"I'm ready only if you are paying my fee for doing this. I suggest that you say a prayer before you enter the court room today cause your case is really weak."

"I thought it was your job to make it strong."

"No lawyer in the world could make your case strong without lying."

"You just better hope I win, if I don't you will have a surprise waiting for you when you get home."

"I don't like threats Mr. Kendricks. I think you should go take a little walk to cool off."

"I think I will do that."

Shawn finally finished the file twenty minutes before court time. Marco came back still being as smart as ever. Shawn had just about had enough of Marco and his cocky attitude.

"Are you ready to fight for your freedom, Marco?"

"Yeah. I'm ready."

All of a sudden the phone rang.

"Hello."

"It's time to come to trial."

"Okay, thank you."

"Marco it's time to go."

10:30. Court was in recess awaiting the judge's decision. Marco was pacing back and forth.

"They nailed me to the wall in there. Do you think I have a chance?"

Shawn really didn't think he would get less then twenty-five years, but since he was his client he had to make it sound good.

"I don't think you are going to have to spend too much time behind bars, but I don't believe you're off the hook."

Marco had an evil look on his face. He wanted out of this as soon as possible.

"When do we go back in?"

"Any minute now we should be able to."

Just then the bailiff came out of the courtroom.

"We are ready to proceed."

Shawn and Marco went back into the courtroom awaiting the judge's decision.

"Okay, gentleman, in the case if Kendricks vs. State my decision goes with the state. Therefore Mr. Kendricks you will be serving a twenty-five year sentence without parole. Sentence starts in two days."

Marco's head dropped. Now all he thought about was revenge.

"Now what, I'm going to jail no thanks to you."

Shawn took a deep breath.

"I did my job as best as I could. The final say is with the judge."

"It's payback time."

Marco stormed out of the courtroom and left Shawn with no explanation.

Shawn headed back to the office to work on his other case. He regretted the fact that he lost Marco's case. He was still trying to figure out what Marco meant by 'payback time'. He knew Marco pretty well and he wouldn't say that unless he meant it. Marco alone was dangerous, but with jail time hanging over his head he was liable to do anything.

At the time, Marco was calling in his hit men.

"Rock at your service."

"Hello, Rock, I have a little job for you."

"What job is that?"

"I want you to hurt someone but I don't want you to kill them."

"No problems give me the address."

"13753 E. Union Drive. You'll find a woman there."

"I'm on my way."

At the same time, Jazmean was working on some paper work. No one was in the store but her and another employee. She had forgotten all about Shawn and his case. She flooded her mind with work related problems and blocked her personal situation out of her mind.

"Hey, Jazmean, I'm headed out to the bank. I'll be back in ten."

"No problem, Todd, I'll be fine."

Five minutes later Rock came in the door.

"Welcome to World Read. Can I help you?"

Rock pulled a gun out of his pocket and pointed it at Jazmean.

"Please don't shoot me."

"Don't worry I won't kill you."

He took the butt of the gun and hit her over the head with it. After that he dragged her behind the counter so that no one would see her. Then he left out the back door.

Todd came back and looked for Jazmean. He couldn't find her anywhere.

"Jazmean, are you still here?"

He walked around the counter and saw her lying on the floor. The first thing he did was call 911 then he called Shawn.

"This is Shawn."

"Shawn, this is Todd. Jazmean's been attacked. I have already called the police and they are on their way."

"Did you see who did it?"

"No. I think you should get here as soon as you can."

"I'm on my way now."

Shawn hung up the phone and rushed out of the office. His boss saw him and tried to stop him.

"Where are you going?"

"I have something important to do. I'll get back when I can."

Shawn rushed past him and out of the door. All he could think about was that Jazmean was pregnant. He didn't know what exactly had happened but he hoped that she would be okay. He ran every red light that he came to and was at the store in ten minutes. Todd was the first person he saw.

"Where is she?"

"Behind the counter."

"The police aren't here yet?"

"No. I don't know what is taking so long."

Shawn bent down to see if she was breathing. She was but she was still unconscious. A few minutes later the ambulance came and took her to the hospital. Shawn was by her side the whole time until the doctors took her in for tests. He prayed to God that she would be okay. In a split second he realized something. *'Its pay back time'* entered his head. Everything after that pointed directly to Marco. Shawn was furious by the time he figured that out. He didn't want to leave Jazmean until he found out she was okay so he stayed. When he heard she was okay he went to see her.

She was unconscious, so he just kissed her head and whispered, "I'll get who ever did this to you. I promise."

In a rage, Shawn left the hospital. He reached under the seat of his car and got the gun that was there. It was the same one that Marco had given him. Shawn thought that if he would have to kill him it would be with his own gun. A few minutes later he was in front of Marco's house. He put the gun in his jacket and walked up to the door.

Knock. Knock.

"Just a minute, here I come."

Marco walked to the door and opened it. The first thing Shawn did was punch him in the face.

"How do you like that? I told you if you messed with Shantell you would have to deal with me. Now you decide to mess with Jazmean you will have to die."

Marco was in shock.

"Wait a minute, man, I didn't do it alone."

"Guess what, smart ass; one thing you didn't know was that Jazmean is pregnant."

Marco had nothing to say. He had really messed up now. He only wanted to get Shawn's attention.

"I'm sorry, Shawn, I didn't know."

"I'll bet you didn't. I better not find out who you hired to do this, because if I do you will have a dead man on your hands."

"You don't have the guts."

Shawn was through listening to Marco's smart mouth. He pulled out the gun and pointed it at Marco.

"*Now* do you think I have the guts?"

Marco was shaking.

"Yeah! Yeah, man! You got the guts."

"Good. If I would have killed you it would have been a suicide. You forgot this is *your* gun."

Shawn dropped the gun on top of Marco's head and

walked out slamming the door behind him. When he was in his car he took a deep breath and cleared his mind for a minute. He couldn't let Jazmean know he went to pay Marco a little visit. Jazmean was too important to him to make her worry more about something like Marco. He finally started the car and drove to the hospital.

"Jazmean, are you awake?"
"Shawn, where have you been?"
"Don't worry about me. Are you okay?"
"I'll fine. Answer my question."
"I went to find out who did this to you."
"Shawn I know it was one of Marco's friends."
Shawn was surprised.
"How do you know?"
"After you left this morning Marco called and said tell your man I'll be waiting for him. I knew there was something fishy about that. I was scared so I left for work and put it out of my mind."
"Why didn't you tell me?"
"I don't know."
"Well, don't worry about it. Marco won't be doing anything else for a long time."
"What did you do?"
"I didn't really do anything. The judge sentenced him to twenty-five years."
"I'm glad he'll be behind bars."
"Jazmean, just forget about Marco. You need to get some rest. I want you out of this hospital soon."
Jazmean took a deep breath and gave Shawn a kiss.
"You need to go home and get some rest, too."
Shawn gave her a kiss in return and went home.

Chapter 11

It was the next morning. After all of the drama of yesterday Shawn was still upset. He hadn't gotten much sleep. He stayed up thinking most of the time. What was really bothering him was that he actually pulled a gun on Marco, and if Marco would have really made him mad he would have shot him. It was a good thing he didn't because he would have to defend *himself* in court. Besides Marco was going to jail and he would pay for what he did anyway.

Another thing that kept Shawn awake was worrying about Jazmean. His girl was pregnant and Marco had the nerve to have someone attack her for his revenge. Jazmean at this point meant the world to him. Now more than ever he would rather it be him in that hospital than Jazmean. Even with all of that; he believed everything was going to be okay.

Twenty minutes later Shawn headed over to the hospital to see Jazmean. Jazmean wasn't in the room she was in the day before. Shawn got worried and asked one of the nurses if they had seen her.

"Excuse me. Have you seen the woman that was in that room?"

"Yes, sir, she was released."

"Who did she leave with?"

The nurse looked at the chart.

"She left with a woman named Shantell."

"Thank you."

Shawn began to ask himself, 'Why didn't she wait for me or at least call?'. He left the hospital and drove over to Shantell's house. He got out of the car ready to get some answers. He went up the stairs and to the door and began to bang on it really hard.

"Shantell, open up! Is Jazmean in there?"

Shantell finally came and opened the door.

"What the hell is wrong with you? You don't need to be coming up to my door banging on it like you on crack. Now get in here before the neighbors see you."

"I'm sorry! Is Jazmean here?"

Shantell rolled her eyes and said.

"What do you think?"

Shawn was already worried enough.

"Don't play games with me just answer my question."

"Yeah, Shawn, she's in the kitchen."

Shawn walked back to the kitchen and stood there for a minute. Jazmean had her back turned to him so she didn't know he was there. Shawn took a deep breath and walked in.

"So, I guess you couldn't tell me that you were leaving the hospital. I went looking for you and *you* were gone."

"Hold up, Shawn, first of all the least you could do is say hello and see if I'm okay. Second, I *thought* you were going to work so I had Shantell come to get me."

Shawn just looked at Jazmean with a look of just pure confusion.

"First off, you must be okay if you walked out of the hospital with Shantell, and second what makes *you* think *I* would go to work when *you* of all people are in a hospital and are pregnant with my baby."

Shawn turns to Shantell.

"Does that make any sense to you?"

Shantell just looked at him and shrugged her shoulders.

"Well, I'm sorry, Shawn. I didn't know you cared that much."

"You just don't know how much I care."

After saying that he starts to turn and walk away.

"Wait a minute. What do you mean by that?"

"You'll find out later tonight. Be home by 7:30. Don't be late."

With that Shawn walks out leaving Jazmean and Shantell wondering.

Jazmean and Shantell look at each other, at the door, then at each other again.

"What was that about? Do I sense your man has a little attitude?"

"I'm not sure, but I know he's up to something."

"What do you think it is?"

"Hopefully he won't do something crazy like jump off the

building to prove he loves me."

Shantell starts to laugh.

"Do you think he's that crazy?"

"Since that was him pounding on that door like that a few minutes ago; yes I do."

"Well, whatever it is I want to see it."

Suddenly the phone rings and Shantell picks it up.

"Hello."

"This is Shawn but don't let Jazmean know you're talking to me."

"Okay."

"Listen to me carefully. I am planning a surprise for Jazmean at my house. I want you and Jose to come."

"What is this for?"

"If I tell you then you will tell Jazmean."

"I won't. Now tell me."

"Forget it. I want this to stay a surprise. Don't say anything to Jazmean."

"Okay fine."

"Be there at 7:30."

Click.

Shantell hangs up the phone and goes back into the kitchen.

"Who was that?"

"Just some one I work with."

"What did they want?"

"Nothing major but I have to leave for a few hours. Can you stay here until I get back?"

"Yeah, I have nothing to do."

Shantell grabbed her keys and walked out the door. She was headed to Jose's house to tell him about this sudden invitation to Shawn's house. It was likely that Jose wouldn't have a problem with going since he had nothing to do that night anyway. Shantell was desperately trying to figure out what Shawn was planning. After the way he acted at her house she was afraid it was something crazy. She would *soon* find out and it would *blow* her mind.

Shantell sat talking to Jose about this *weird* situation.

"So, what does Shawn plan to do?"

"Beats me, all he told me was that he was planning a surprise for Jazmean and that he wanted us to be there."

"It sounds strange to me, too, but we might as well go."

"We *are* going. I want to see what all of this is about."

"Then it's settled we are going. What time?"

"7:30. One more thing, you will have to drive your car because I have to take Jazmean to pick up her car and I don't want her to be suspicious."

"That's cool with me."

Meanwhile, Shawn was at home about to call Andre. 'This is going to be a night to remember', Shawn thought to himself. Shawn picked up the phone and dialed Andre's number.

"Hello. Andre here."

"Andre, this is Shawn."

"Hey, Shawn, it's good that you called. What's up?"

"Well, you know how I said you could come to dinner one of these days?"

"Yeah. I'm looking forward to that."

"Well, that day is today. I am planning a surprise for Jazmean and I want you and Crystal to be there."

"That's great timing. Crystal is in town for tonight then she's leaving tomorrow."

"Great. Come around 7:30 and be ready for a surprise."

"What is the surprise?"

"You'll have to wait until tonight."

"Okay, we'll be there."

The next thing Shawn had to do was order food. He definitely wasn't going to be cooking. Six people were a lot of people for him to cook for.

"I'll leave the cooking to the pros", he thought to himself.

"Hello."

"Yes, Is this Shay LaReinz? I would like to order a dinner for six to go, please."

"What would you like, sir?"

"Give me the house special."

"Okay, thank you, sir. It will be ready for you by 3:00."

"Thank you."

Now everything was almost setup for his surprise. He still had one more thing to do.

3 o'clock. Shawn is getting ready to leave the house when the phone rings.

"Hello?"

"Shawn, this is Jazmean."

"Hey, baby, what's up?"

"Shawn, I can't stand waiting to see what the surprise is. Can you just tell me?"

Shawn laughs.

"Then it wouldn't be a secret. Listen you only have... four hours until you can find out what the secret is. Until then I am not going to tell you."

Jazmean was getting pretty frustrated about Shawn not telling her about what he was planning.

"Just one little hint?"

"Okay...uh...let's just say it's something that could change your life forever if you accept it. Now I'm not going to say anything else until later."

Just then, someone came knocking on the door.

"Shawn, I've got to go. Someone's at the door. Don't forget I'm not through with you yet."

"Okay, Jaz, I won't."

Shawn hangs up the phone. At the same time, Jazmean was going to answer the door.

"Who's there?"

"It's Teresa."

Jazmean sighed and opened the door.

"How did you know I was here?"

"The nurse at the hospital told me. Anyway I just came to see how you were doing."

"Let me guess...mom sent you."

"You should know that, but I didn't come just because she wanted me to."

"Well, why *did* you come?"

"I came to see if you needed me to do anything for you."

"Well, come to think of it, I do need someone to take me to

the bookstore to get my car."

"Okay, we can go now."

"Let me get my keys and I'll be right there."

Meanwhile, at Shay LaReinz, Shawn was picking up the wonderful food he had ordered for dinner. It was ten till four and he still had one more place to go, the jewelry store. He jumped in his car and rode over to the jewelry store on 119th and Brimstone. It would be closing soon so he would have to hurry.

Shawn got there thirty minutes before closing and he was so glad. A jeweler came over to help him.

"Hello, sir, is there anything I can interest you in this evening?"

"As a matter of fact, you can. Would you happen to have a fourteen karat gold engagement ring with a ten karat diamond?"

The jeweler's eyes got wide at the fact that Shawn knew exactly what he wanted.

"Yes, we happen to have two of them right here."

Shawn looked them both over and made up his mind.

"I'll take that one right there."

"Okay, sir that will be one hundred seventy-five dollars."

This was going to be the only time he would buy a ring for Jazmean so he was going to make the best of it.

"How much is the other one?"

"It is three hundred, sir."

"I'll take it."

Shawn paid for the ring, in cash, and left the store proud to be able to spend that much money.

When he got home he prepared one more surprise for Jazmean. He had bought her a dress a couple of weeks ago and she never found out about it. He decided to make it a surprise for her when she got home. Shawn knew in his mind he couldn't make this anymore special then it already was.

At the time, Jazmean was at World Read picking up her car.

"Thank you so much, Teresa, you have really been a big help."

"It's no problem. You don't have to thank me. I'm your

sister; I'm supposed to help you."

"Well, thanks anyway. I'm heading back to Shantell's, is there anything else you came to see me for?"

"No. I just wanted to check on you."

"All right well, I'll see you later then."

Jazmean hopped in her car and sped off as she usually did when she had somewhere to be.

The time was drawing near for Jazmean's *big* surprise. No one knew what it was except for Shawn and he was keeping it that way. The big moment was going to be Shawn's chance to prove to everyone, including himself, that he *really* loves Jazmean. Little does he know he is going to have a surprise of his own.

Chapter 12

Click. Click. Click.

"Shawn, I'm…………"

Jazmean couldn't even finish her sentence. The room in front of her had been completely transformed into a sophisticated but charming restaurant scene. As she stepped in the door Shawn came out dressed in a suave blue suit that almost made him look like a movie star.

Shawn walked into the room smoothly and said, "Come on in, Jaz, your first surprise is waiting for you in the bedroom."

Without even asking any questions Jazmean went into the bedroom. She was still speechless over Shawn and what he had done to the apartment. When she walked into the bedroom music was playing, candles were lit and there were rose pedals leading to the bed. Overwhelmed she followed the trail and there lay a note on the bed. Underneath it was a dazzling royal blue dress with silver sparkles down the front. Jazmean began to read the note.

"My precious Jazmean,
I hope you like your first surprise. I can't wait to see you in it. There is still more to come so get dressed and meet me in the living room.
Tenderly, Shawn."

By now Jazmean was more ready than ever to see what else Shawn had waiting for her. She wanted to know so many things like; why is he doing this? What will he come up with next? All of that and more was running through her head.

Fifteen minutes later Jazmean came out into the living room. Shawn was waiting for her.

"I see you look as fine as I imagined you would in that dress."

Jazmean finally got up the nerve to say something.

"You look good yourself in that suit."

Shawn took her hand and directed her to her seat.

"Have a seat and let's talk."

Jazmean sat down and Shawn sat beside her.

"So, what kind of impression did you get when you walked in and saw all of this?"

"I wasn't quite sure I was in the right place until I saw you. Then I started to wonder if it was really you. This all feels like a dream."

Shawn smiled a crafty smile.

"Believe me this is no dream, but it will feel more like one later on."   Jazmean was anxious to find out what this whole thing was all about.

"Shawn, can you tell me what is behind all of this?"

Shawn pretended to not know what she meant by that.

"What do you mean?"

"I mean, why are you doing all of this? What are you trying to do?"

"I can only tell you that soon you will love me for what is going to happen tonight."

"That is what I want to know. What is going to happen tonight?"

It was getting harder and harder for Shawn to keep his secret, but he had to until his friends got there.

"Are you thirsty?"

"Yes, but...nevermind go ahead."

Shawn came back with two glasses of sparkling cider and a sly smile on his face.

"When are you going to tell me what is going on?"

Riinngg.

"Maybe I'll do it after I answer the phone."

"Hello."

"Shawn this is Shantell. Is Jazmean there?"

"Yes. She can't wait to find out what my surprise is all about. Where are you?"

"I'm at home and I'm waiting on Jose to get here."

"Well, you two get here as fast as you can. I don't know how long she will wait."

"I will."

Shawn hung up the phone. Jazmean was still sitting in the living room trying to figure out what Shawn was up to, so Shawn picked up the phone and called Andre.

Ring. Ring. Ring.

"Hello."
"Hey, Andre, this is Shawn."
"Oh, I thought it was someone else. What's up?"
"Are you and Crystal still coming?"
"Yeah. We'll be there in about ten minutes."
"Okay, that's cool. I'll see you then."
Click.
"Shawn, who were you just talking to a second ago?"
Jazmean had walked in right after Shawn hung up the phone.
"I was talking to one of our guests. You don't need to worry everything is going just as planned."
"That is what I am afraid of, Shawn. I don't know..."
Knock. Knock.
"That may be one of our guests right now."
"Shawn, I'm not to sure about this."
"Trust me."
Shawn goes and answers the door as if to make the whole situation more dramatic.
"Hello. I'm glad you made it."
"We are glad to be here."
"Go on in and have a seat."
When Shantell and Jose walk in, and Jazmean sees them, she gets even more suspicious.
"Shawn, can I speak to you for a minute?"
"Just one minute, Jaz, I'll be right there."
"Make yourselves at home and don't worry about Jazmean she...."
There was a knock at the door.
"Shantell, could you get that for me?"
"No problem."
When Shantell answered the door it was Andre and Crystal.
"Andre, please come in. I will be right back," Shawn said trying to go talk to Jazmean.
Jazmean had gone back into the bedroom. Shawn went back there to talk to her hoping that he hadn't made her mad.
"Jazmean, did you want something?"
"Yes, Shawn, I want to know what this is all about."

Shawn was tired of keeping his secret but he had to keep it for a few more minutes.

"Jazmean, I don't mean to cut you off, but I will be right back and I promise I will give you an answer."

Shawn hurried back into the living room and to the kitchen. He pulled his wonderfully prepared feast out of the oven and took it to the dining room.

"Ladies and gentlemen, in a few moments you will all get to enjoy this food and find out why you are really here, but until then you can admire the wonderful food. I will be back in a moment."

Shawn walked back into the bedroom to see Jazmean exactly as he left her, confused.

"Now, Jazmean, I invited your friends and mine to dinner because I have something that I want to share with you and I want them to witness it."

"What is it? I have been waiting and I still don't know."

Shawn grinned making fun of Jazmean's intensity.

"Well, you will wait no longer. Close your eyes and let me guide you to the dining room."

Jazmean did as she was told and Shawn led her to their waiting guests.

"Now open your eyes."

When Jazmean opened her eyes she saw all the wonderful food and her friends sitting at the table, which almost made her cry.

Shawn was ready to make his announcement, but he wasn't sure everyone else was ready.

"Before we eat, I would like to let you all witness why we are all here. To make this short I'm going to say that my heart is racing and I'm not sure about this."

He turns to Jazmean who is just waiting to hear what he has to say.

"Jazmean, we have been together almost six months now, and you are carrying my child, and I couldn't be happier. There is only a small piece missing from the whole puzzle. That piece is the one I want to put in place tonight."

Everyone, including Jazmean, is listening intently to

what Shawn is saying, but none of them have caught on. Shawn takes Jazmean's hand and bends down to one knee.

"Jazmean, I love you with all my heart and here tonight I want to give you my heart to keep forever. I want you to give me the pleasure of fulfilling my dreams tonight. Jazmean, will you marry me?"

No one in the room can say a word. Shawn looks into Jazmean's eyes with complete sincerity and waits for an answer.

"I...I...Yes...Yes, Shawn, I will marry you."

Shawn stands up from his one knee and gives Jazmean a kiss.

"Thank you, Jazmean you have just completed my life."

Shantell, Jose, Andre, and Crystal all stand and give Shawn and Jazmean a round of applause. Shawn takes a deep breath and tries to speak.

"Now, all of you know why I asked you all to come here. I am about to start spending the rest of my life with a very wonderful woman. Now that that's done let's celebrate with some food."

The dinner continues to go wonderfully and they all get to talking and getting to know each other better. Jazmean and Shawn were in the spotlight the whole night and they didn't even mind. Shawn was happy for the first time in a long time. He finally had what he really wanted in a woman.

It was after everyone had left that everything had started to sink in. Jazmean was sitting by the window, like she had done before, looking out over Lake Michigan. She really loved Shawn, but now she had said yes to spend the rest of her life with him. She hated to say it, but she was having second thoughts. Shawn had walked into the room and seen the tears falling from her eyes and knew something was wrong.

"Jaz, what's wrong?"

All she could do was fall into his arms.

"You don't have to tell me. I get the feeling that you are having second thoughts about us."

Jazmean looked up into Shawn's eyes with sadness.

"I do love you, but I just don't know if we should even think about getting married."

Shawn closed his eyes. He was truly hurt by what Jazmean felt.

"I knew this would happen. I tried to block it out of my mind. At the moment I asked you I knew you wouldn't turn me down, but I knew afterwards you would think back on it and have second thoughts."

"Shawn it's not that at all. I..."

"Don't, Jazmean. Let's just go to sleep in each others arms and just think of the good side. We still have tomorrow. We can take it one day at a time."

Jazmean fell asleep in Shawn's arms as she had done before, but this time Shawn was awake wondering if he had made a mistake and done things *too soon*. He was not even going to think about that. The next day would be just like the day before. Too soon wasn't even soon enough.

The End

About the Author

Marquita, a very bright young lady, enjoys writing stories that can influence the lives of others. This book was written to get the reader thinking about their own life and how it relates to the life of the character. This book is meant to put the reader right into the story.

Marquita, born in Kansas City, Missouri in 1983, has accomplished a lot in her life. This being her first book she enjoys the comments she gets about the ending. The sequel to this book, A Second Chance, is just as interesting as this one with scenes that make you turn the page really quickly. For more of Marquita's work explore her wonderful collection that will blow your mind.

CPSIA information can be obtained at www.ICGtesting.com
Printed in the USA
BVOW072045211211

278904BV00001B/3/P